I0436295

CHRONIC DISEASES'
BEST NATUROPATHIC ADVICE *

TO HELP& PREVENT:
1) ARTHRITIS 2) BREAST CANCER
3) PROSTATE CANCER
4) CROHN'S 5) The Common COLD.

Written by: SHEILA BER – Naturopathic Consultant.

INTRODUCTION:

I'm a Microbiological/Chemical Technologist, who is currently working as a Naturopathic Consultant.

I'm writing this book to provide advice to help and prevent, several chronic diseases, that I have experienced myself. I'm a survivor of Breast Cancer, Crohn's disease, as well as of Arthritis.

Much of the advice provided in this book, is also from my microbiological and chemical background knowledge and experience.

I'm a successful survivor of Breast cancer, Crohn's disease, and Arthritis.

I dedicate the book to my sons: Philip and Bernard. The book is also dedicated to all who seek help, for their unnecessary pain and suffering.

INDEX:

What is pH?

pH is an acronym for the "potential of Hydrogen", or the acid to alkaline ratio existing in all matter, and our 7.365 body pH measurement is the benchmark for measuring our health. Our pH normal range value can be likened to our body's temperature; we each have a normal range value of 98.6 degrees. When our body temperature increases or decreases we typically experience symptoms, and more importantly, we also know there is an underlying reason when our temperature is not normal.

pH scale measures acid to alkaline: 0 to 14.
Our body pH should be 7.365, which is considered neutral.

7.365 being neutral, if your pH is 6.365 - you are 10x more acidic than normal range.

7.365 being neutral, if your pH is 5.365 - you are 100x more acidic than normal range.

You can see how the pH factor compounds itself. This is why people will feel as though their health has spiraled, and thus are required to take action to normalize their pH balance.

ALKALIZE and SURVIVE! - *See how on page #11.*

BREAST CANCER PREVENTION TIPS AND ADVICE by SHEILA BER (survivor) & Naturopathic Consultant.

50% OF ALL CANCERS CAN BE PREVENTED!

1) *ALKALIZE YOUR BODY* –The simplest, economical way to alkalize: 1/2 tsp Baking Soda (Arm & Hammer brand) in 1 cup water, daily, along with 1 Potassium tablet 99 mg. in order to keep the Sodium Potassium ratio balanced.
2) *TAKE DAILY VITAMIN D3*, 5,000-10,000 I.U. divided in 2: am & pm. I take 5,000 I.U. twice a day. It keeps me in Optimum health.

If your diet consists of excessive carbohydrates (including sugars), and your stress level is very high, you take medication, you smoke, your body pH would definitely be very acidic.

You then have to take Baking soda, 2x a day, to ensure your body is NOT ACIDIC, so that it will discourage CANCER from thriving.

Note: CANCER CELLS love to thrive in an acidic environment only.

It is basic chemistry!

2) Take PROBIOTICS: 1-2 capsules a day.

3) Eat plenty of fruits and vegetables. Less Carbohydrates and fats.

4) Take 1-2 tablespoon Flax oil, and/or Cod liver fish oil daily! They reduce inflammation, and also lower the risk for cancer.

5) Don't smoke, nor eat smoked foods. Stay away from meats such as cold cuts. Eat fish, chicken and legumes that have cancer fighting properties.

6) Use toothpastes that are Fluoride and Paraben free. Fluoride competes with the Iodine in your body, thus causing thyroid and hormones' imbalance.

7) Use cleaning agents that are green and free of volatile harmful chemicals.

8) To replace deodorants: use a small mixture of <u>baking soda</u> and water, and apply under arms etc.

It will keep you smelling fresh for several days. You can repeat daily. It is cheap, effective and simple.
It does not leave stains on your clothing.

9) Refrain from drinking alcohol, if possible. Alcohol raises Estrogen level, fuelling cancer growth, (especially hormonal cancer) if excessive.

10) Check periodically your thyroid level. The Thyroid controls all bodily functions, including hormones.

11) All alcoholic drinks contain yeast. Yeast overgrowth is toxic, damaging, and can make you prone to cancer.

When you eat or drink yeasty foods, drinks, such as: PIZZA, PASTRY, WINE, BEER, consume in moderation, and immediately take Probiotics, to get rid of the excessive yeast in your body.

 Probiotics also digest and kill yeast.

*Please note: A strong presence of Yeast/Candida can pose a high risk of developing breast cancer.

12) Daily check your urine pH level. Optimum pH is (6.5-7.5).

13) Do blood test, once in 6 months, and check your ESR level (Erythrocyte Sedimentation Rate).
 It indicates the inflammation rate in your body. High inflammation level can induce cancer growth. Check also your _liver_ status.

14) Check your <u>hormones</u> level. If your Estrogen level is high, you are then considered to be Estrogen dominant, and therefore, at a greater risk of developing hormonally associated cancer.
<u>To balance your hormones</u>, it is recommended to use Bioidentical Progesterone cream 3%-6%, once or 2x daily. You simply apply it on the skin, daily, alternating areas: <u>abdomen</u>, <u>front neck</u>, <u>inside mid-arms</u>, <u>inside and back of thighs</u>.

You'll require a Doctor's prescription. Any Dr. with an alternative approach will be happy to assist you. Bioidentical Progesterone is beneficial for: Thyroid balance, bone health, heart health, nervous system and much more.

For more information go to:

<u>http://www.hystersisters.com/vb2/article_97232.htm</u>
and
<u>http://www.hormone-healthy.com/Benefits_of_Natural_Progesterone.htm</u>.

15) Check with a Naturopathic Doctor, whether you have parasites, particularly the FLUKES, that cause cancer! The test is brief and simple, and it's done through <u>Electro Dermal sensors' computerized device.</u>

*I had breast cancer, and found out through this test, that I had Flukes that took over, nearly 70% of my body, when the cancer was already present. Had I known earlier, that I had them, and got an adequate treatment, cancer would not have been the result.

You can get Flukes, by eating vegetables, improperly washed, also fish and meat insufficiently cooked.

16) Keep your stress level down. Find ways to deal with it effectively, so that it won't leave negative, toxic impact on your body, that can result in cancer, or in other serious illnesses.

<u>Body chemistry:</u> Stress, acidic diet, medications, alcohol, cigarette smoking, parasites (including yeast, fungus), all contribute to acidic body pH.

It is extremely difficult to stay slightly alkaline at all times, for most people, unless one takes action to reverse the acidic pH.

HOW TO ALKALIZE – TO BALANCE YOUR pH.

Simplest way to reverse acidity is to alkalize: drink 1/2 teaspoon BAKING SODA in 1 cup water, with 1 POTASSIUM tablet (to keep your electrolytes balanced). Do it 1-2 a day. Baking Soda is harmless, provides you with energy, added Oxygen, better digestion, has detoxifying effect, and neutralizes your body acidity.

If your acidity level is much too high, you need to repeat the above 2-3 times a day, so that your body will be slightly alkaline: pH 7.0-7.5.
**To test your blood pH, you simply check the pH in your urine, 1-2 times a day. If you have cancer, you need to check at least 3x a day. Cancer further acidifies the body, by releasing its toxins.

A simple test is done with a Q-Tip (coated with Turmeric, and has light yellow color) and is placed under the stream of urine.

If the pH is acidic, it will remain yellow, and if it is alkaline, the color of the Q-Tip will appear in color ranging from orange to red wine.
Orange to red wine, are the colors that you want to attain. If you see yellow on your Q-tip, immediately alkalize, by taking your Baking Soda drink, as described above.

***To prepare your Q-Tips for the test, do the following simple steps: In a small container, place several tablespoons of rubbing Ethyl alcohol (Pharmacy). Mix in: 1/2 teaspoon Turmeric powder. Mix well. Immerse 10-20 Q-Tips in the mixture. Let dry over a piece of paper. Cut them in 1/2, so you can use both ends for more tests. You'll have a month supply to do your daily pH tests.*

17) You must take your <u>daily vitamins</u> and minerals that help combat cancer, and the most important ones are:

BETA CAROTENE - 20,000 I.U.

B-12 - <u>Methylcobalamin</u> version is best! For optimum absorption, 1000-5000 mcg.

FOLIC ACID - 5 mg.

MULTI-VITAMINS & MINERALS.

B-COMPLEX 50-100 mg..

VITAMIN C - 2,000 mg.

Most important Minerals: Zinc Citrate - 100 mg. Selenium - 100 - 200 mcg, Potassium 99 mg, Calcium Citrate 1000mg - 1200 mg. daily, Magnesium Citrate/Malate 500 mg.

18) You must also take Pancreatic enzymes containing Ox bile. Enzymes digest food, parasites, cancer cells, putrid matter left in the bowels. They help break it down, and keep the body clean. It also helps in reducing inflammation. Take one with every meal.

It is also recommended to take 2 tablets before going to bed at night. If you have cancer, take up to 5 enzyme tablets nightly, as enzymes help digest cancer cells.

I hope you find the above information helpful to you.

SHEILA BER, 2012.

Disclaimer.

Copyright © 2012 Sheila Ber. All rights reserved.

PROSTATE CANCER PREVENTION TIPS AND ADVICE.

50% OF ALL CANCERS CAN BE PREVENTED!

1) *ALKALIZE YOUR BODY* –The simplest, economical way to alkalize: 1/2 tsp Baking Soda (Arm & Hammer brand) in 1 cup water, daily, along with 1 Potassium tablet 99 mg. in order to keep the Sodium Potassium ratio balanced.
 2) *TAKE DAILY VITAMIN D3*, 5,000-10,000 I.U. divided in 2: am & pm. I take 5,000 I.U. twice a day. It keeps me in Optimum health.

If your diet consists of excessive carbohydrates (including Sugars), and your stress level is very high, you take medication, and/or you smoke, consequently your body pH would definitely be highly acidic.

Easiest way to neutralize it, is by taking the basic alkalizer, Baking Soda. Take it 2x a day, to ensure your body is NOT ACIDIC, so that it discourages CANCER from thriving, and/or spreading. Note: CANCER CELLS love to thrive in an acidic environment only.

It is basic chemistry!

2) Take PROBIOTICS: 1-2 capsules a day.

3) Eats plenty of fruits and vegetables. Less Carbohydrates and fats.

4) Take 1-2 tablespoon Flax oil/Cod liver fish oil daily! They reduce inflammation, thus also lower the risk for cancer.

5) Don't smoke, nor eat smoked foods. Stay away from meat cold cuts. Eat fish, chicken and legumes that have cancer fighting properties.

6) *Use toothpastes that are <u>Fluoride and Paraben free.</u> Fluoride competes with the Iodine in your body, thus causing thyroid and hormones' imbalance.*

7) *Use cleaning agents that are green and free of volatile harmful chemicals.*

8) *To replace deodorants: use a small mixture of <u>baking soda</u> and water, and apply under arms etc.*
It will keep you smelling fresh for several days. You can repeat daily. It is cheap, effective and simple.
It does not leave stains on your clothing.

9) *Refrain from drinking alcohol, if possible. Alcohol raises Estrogen level, provoking and fuelling cancer growth, (especially hormonal cancer) if consumed excessively.*

10) *Check periodically your thyroid level. The Thyroid controls all bodily functions, including hormones.*

11) *All alcoholic drinks contain yeast. Yeast overgrowth is toxic, damaging, and can make you prone to cancer.*

When you eat or drink yeasty foods, drinks, such as: PIZZA, PASTRY, WINE, BEER, consume in moderation, and immediately take Probiotics, to get rid of the excessive yeast in your body. Probiotics also digest and kill yeast.

*Please note: A strong presence of Yeast/Candida can pose a high risk of developing Prostate cancer.

12) Daily check your urine pH level. Optimum pH is: (6.5-7.5).

13) Do blood test, once in 6 months, and check your ESR level (Erythrocyte Sedimentation Rate).
It indicates the inflammation rate in your body. High inflammation level can induce cancer growth. Check also your liver status.

14) Check your hormones level. If your Estrogen level is high, you are then considered to be Estrogen dominant, and therefore, at a greater risk of developing hormonally associated cancer.
To balance your hormones, it is recommended to use Bioidentical Progesterone cream 3%-6%, once or 2x daily.

Indeed, Bio-identical Progesterone (natural source) is also prescribed for men. It reduces Estrogen dominance, by balancing in the most natural and efficient manner, the Estrogen/Progesterone ratio, without any side effects.

You simply apply it on the skin, daily alternating areas: abdomen, front neck, inside mid-arms, inside and back of thighs.

You'll require a Doctor's prescription. Any Dr. with an alternative approach will be happy to assist.

Bioidentical Progesterone is beneficial for: Thyroid balance, bone health, heart health, nervous system and much more.

For more information go to:

http://www.hystersisters.com/vb2/article_97232.htm
and
http://www.hormone-healthy.com/Benefits_of_Natural_Progesterone.htm.

15) Check with a Naturopathic Doctor, whether you have parasites, particularly the FLUKES, that cause cancer! The test is brief and simple, and it's done through Electro Dermal sensors' computerized device.

*I had breast cancer, and found out through this test, that I had Flukes that took over, nearly 70% of my body, when the cancer was already present. Had I known earlier, that I had them, and got an adequate treatment, cancer would not have been the result.

You can get Flukes, by eating vegetables, improperly washed, also fish and meat insufficiently cooked.

*Please note: Prostate cancer is a hormonal cancer, and its causes are in many ways similar to female hormonal cancers.

16) Keep your stress level down. Find ways to deal with it effectively, so that it won't leave a negative, toxic impact on your body, which may result in cancer, or in other serious illness.

Body chemistry: Stress, acidic diet, medications, alcohol, cigarette smoking, parasites (including yeast, fungus), all contribute to acidic body pH.

It is extremely difficult to stay slightly alkaline at all times, for most people, unless one takes action to reverse the acidic body pH. Simplest way to alkalize is to: drink 1/2 teaspoon BAKING SODA (Arm & Hammer brand) in 1 cup water, with 1 POTASSIUM tablet 99 mg. (to keep your electrolytes balanced). Do it 1-2 a day.

Baking Soda is harmless, provides you with energy, added Oxygen, better digestion, has detoxifying effect, and neutralizes your body acidity.
If your acidity level is much too high, you need to repeat the above 2-3 times a day, so that you will maintain your body slightly alkaline: pH 7.0-7.5.

**To test your blood pH, you simply check the pH in your urine, 1-2 times a day. If you have cancer, you need to check at least 3x a day. Cancer further acidifies the body, by releasing its toxins.

A simple test is done with a Q-Tip (coated with Turmeric, and has light yellow color) and is placed under the stream of urine.

If the pH is acidic, it will remain yellow, and if it is alkaline, the color of the Q-Tip will appear in color ranging from orange to red wine.

Orange to red wine, are the colors that you want to get. If you see yellow on your Q-tip, immediately alkalize, by taking your Baking Soda drink, as described above.

**To prepare your Q-Tips for the test, do the following simple steps: In a small container, place several tablespoons of rubbing Ethyl alcohol (Pharmacy). Mix in: 1/2 teaspoon Turmeric powder. Mix well. Immerse 10-20 Q-Tips in the mixture. Let dry over a piece of paper. Cut them in 1/2, so you can use both ends for more tests. You'll have a month supply to do your daily pH tests.

17) You must take your <u>daily:</u>
 vitamins and minerals that help combat cancer, and the most important ones are:

BETA CAROTENE - 20,000 I.U.

B-12 - Methyl cobalamin version is best! For optimum absorption, 1000-5000 mcg.

FOLIC ACID - 5 mg.

MULTI-VITAMINS & MINERALS.

B-COMPLEX 50-100 mg.

VITAMIN C - 2,000 mg.

Most important Minerals:

Zinc Citrate - 100 mg.
Selenium - 100 - 200 mcg, Potassium 99 mg, Calcium Citrate 1000mg - 1200 mg. daily, Magnesium Citrate/Malate 500 mg.

18) You must also take Pancreatic enzymes containing Ox bile. Enzymes digest food, parasites, cancer cells, putrid matter left in the bowels. They help break it down, and keep the body clean. It also helps in reducing inflammation.

Take one with every meal.

It is also recommended to take 2 tablets before going to bed at night. If you have cancer, take up to 5 enzyme tablets nightly, as enzymes help digest cancer cells.

SHEILA BER, 2012.

Disclaimer.

Copyright © 2012 Sheila Ber. All rights reserved.

CROHN'S DISEASE HELP and BEST ADVICE – My Personal Successful Regimen.

MY BEST ADVICE TO YOU:

Vitamin D3 *deficiency is a major factor for Crohn's. I take 8,000 - 10,000 I.U. a day, divided by two, 2x a day.*

Try like myself taking the above dosage, but always with a spoon of Flax or Fish oil, to optimize absorption. Vitamin D will give you energy, reduce inflammation, balance your Thyroid, and other hormones, protect you against developing cancer, maintain healthy nervous system, help you sleep better, and much more.

Eliminate sugars and replace with Honey in everything! Honey is comprised of mono-saccharides, and easily digested by Crohn's afflicted bowels, therefore less bacterial growth that causes inflammation. Try also to take 1/2 tsp of MANUKA HONEY, on empty stomach 1 hour before a meal. Manuka addresses pain and inflammation in a very natural, simple and efficient way, almost like magic. Use it daily!

This honey heals any wound inside and outside the body!!!
<u>If you are allergic to fructose, do not eat honey!</u> Try Stevia. MANUKA honey is a product of New Zealand.

* Please note: If honey isn't stored properly, or comes in an inadequate packaging, it is vulnerable to bacterial contamination. It may be stored at room temperature, always with the lid properly closed.

It helps against any abdominal pain! I tried it when I had pain from Crohn's attack, the pain was gone. The cost is about $15.00 for small jar, and it lasts for a reasonably long time.

SUGAR- IN ANY FORM, IS EXTREMELY HARMFUL TO THE INFLAMED BOWELS OF CROHN'S SUFFERERS.

Try to avoid smoking, and coffee, only once a day or every other day!

Instead of coffee, to be alert and awake, put a dash or two of CAYENNE PEPPER into 1/2 cup of warm water, or into salads, soups, any dishes. It does wonders! It also takes pain away!!!

Taking daily: 2 Tablespoons of APPLE CIDER VINEGAR in 1 cup of warm water, helps tremendously. Absolutely!

I take also 1 coated baby Aspirin 81 mg. every day, or every other day. It keeps inflammation down, and the blood thin, due to high ESR associated with Crohn's disease.
It prevents potential strokes in older adults, due to associated high blood Platelets count, and high ESR (Erythrocyte Sedimentation Rate).

You will not regret implementing the above suggestions, as you are getting them from a Crohn's sufferer like yourself, who is mature in years, and with experience, and who has tried everything. I have provided in this book, many helpful suggestions for emergency situations. If you don't try, you'll never know...

Check with your G.P. your thyroid level, and Hemoglobin level as well. You might need Iron pills (best from vegetable source). www.vitacost.com sells them at a reasonable price –
Item #CTL4026594. Take 3 a day with vitamin C- 500-1000 mg. for about 3 months.

When in intense pain, for immediate relief, take also 1 tablespoon Colloidal Silver, but swash in the mouth for a few seconds, then swallow. In 5-7 minutes, the pain subsides.

Additionally take: <u>***ROBERT'S COMPLEX***</u> *Enzymatic therapy (Approx. $20.00), which is extremely helpful to avert an attack.*

Take it 3x a day, for several days only, on an empty stomach until you feel better.

Crohn's pain, any abdominal pain, can be alleviated effectively also, with boiled (5 min.) herbal concoction: Sage, Mint, Anise. Drink warm, several times/day. It's very healing and detoxifying. Don't forget the MANUKA HONEY also for the pain!

<u>***Don't:***</u> *eat fried food!*

<u>Don't drink raw milk!</u> You must minimize drinking milk. You can drink 2-3 cups a week, but <u>you must boil it first!!!</u> Because milk has a specific bacteria that aggravates severely the Crohn's, but if you boil it, you should have no problem.

<u>Do not</u> drink alcohol, as all alcoholic drinks contain yeast. Yeast overgrowth is toxic, damaging, and can cause inflammation.

7a) When you eat or drink <u>yeasty foods, drinks</u>, such as: PIZZA, PASTRY, WINE, BEER, consume in moderation, and immediately take Probiotics, to get rid of the yeast in your body, before it gets out of control. Probiotics also digest and kill yeast.

<u>Do eat</u>: 2-3x a week SALMON fish, and also chicken. These are healing to the bowels, and anti-inflammatory. They are beneficial for the heart, brain, and for depression as well.

Take: Cod liver oil: 2-3 tablespoons daily. It is anti inflammatory, and keeps your blood vessels in good shape. It also helps ward off depression.

Eat rice daily if you can, until you get better. When you feel better, you can increase your potatoes and bread (whole wheat or 7 grains) intake. Rice is the only complex carbs that really best agrees with Crohn's. You can cook it in many ways.

You can even add raisins, silvered almonds, add 3 tablespoons of honey, 2 tablespoon Grape seed oil (best oil) and 1/2 teaspoon butter, nutmeg, some cinnamon, grated lemon peel (1/3 teaspoon), 1/2 cup milk, or condensed milk (in a can). Bring to a boil, and simmer for about 15 minutes. Eat cool or warm.

The worst thing that you can do is to feel sorry for yourself. I know Crohn's can cause depression. But you have to remain strong, positive, and hopeful! You must move on with life.

You have to be flexible when it comes to food, and give up the items that cause you trouble (inflammation).

*If you make a mistake and you eat something you shouldn't, or if stress causes you an attack, despite all efforts, don't give up! Keep fighting it, and do all the tips given to you in this book.

It takes time to heal, and slowly you will heal, I promise! However, you have to make some changes, you just have to, or you could suffer big time.

Try and visualize your intestines, and what you put into them!

Always take HONEY to substitute sugar! Also MANUKA HONEY for <u>pain</u>. Take also PROBIOTICS ("Primal Defense" is best!) to keep microbial level, and inflammation down.

If you are allergic to fructose, do not eat honey!

Remember that the intestines can heal at any moment, slowly and surely.

However, you have to control what you eat, and how much. Again, just try to look inside you. Stay calm, and try not to worry. Worries, stress, definitely aggravate Crohn's.

If you feel depressed, you must take B-Complex 2-3 times a day, and L-Theanine (amino acid) 1-2 capsules a day. Drink coffee, no more than once a day, as it can aggravate the inflammation in your bowels. However, at the same time, it is beneficial in elevating your Serotonin level, making you feeling content).

To fight depression and inflammation, take also 2 tablespoon cod liver oil daily. The oil is extremely helpful, and has many health benefits. It contains Vitamin A&D, also EPA and DHA.

If you fancy Chinese food, it can be oily.
Vegies and rice, that are not oily, are OK. Soya sauce can aggravate Crohn's, so try to stay away from it.

Orange is also very aggravating. Instead of lemon use lime, as it feels better for the Crohn's bowels.

Chicken Teriyaki has soya sauce and it can aggravate. Steak is good, potatoes I find OK, with added olive oil over them, some parsley, lime juice and salt, it's all healing and excellent tasting.

<u>Eggs</u>- I find that if you eat them 3 times a week, and then rest 2-3 days, alternately, your body is less likely to develop intolerance (allergy) for eggs. But then it is individual.

White flour in any form or shape (bread, cakes, cookies etc) can be harmful for Crohn's. I eat whole wheat bread, or 7 grains, but keep it to minimum, because the flour converts to sugars (polysaccharides and disaccharides,) and the bowels have difficult time digesting them.

Complex Carbs such as rice is all right. (Basmati is best!). Potatoes, are all right, if eaten 2-3 times a week. Due to their high starch content, the bowels can have difficult time digesting them.

Sandwich with home cooked meat is OK, but definitely <u>not the cold cuts</u>! Cold cuts will cause an immediate attack, and more inflammation as a result. The bowels can react very negatively, including the forming intestinal blockage. The preservatives in the cold cuts: Sodium Nitrate & Sodium Nitrite, are carcinogenic, and are also very aggravating to the Crohn's afflicted bowels.

<u>Don't eat</u>: Oranges, lemons, chocolate or pizza, as they can induce an attack due to irritability of the small bowels. When you feel better you may gradually introduce them to your diet.

*Personally, I can never eat an orange, but
I can have a few drops of lemon in a glass of water, before
breakfast, to maintain optimum liver health.*

*<u>Do eat</u>: Bananas (excellent! even 2-3x a day), broccoli is very
good, but must be washed and boiled for 3-5 minutes, to make
it easier on the bowels to digest. Carrots are very good, but
until your bowels get better, you must cook the carrots for
about 10 minutes, for easier digestion.*

*Tomatoes are very good, but can irritate your sensitive bowels.
You may eat fresh tomatoes with sprinkled Olive oil on top.
It tastes great. The Olive oil coats the bowels, preventing the
acidity from the tomatoes from interacting with them.*

*Pizza - 1-2 slices are OK, but because of the <u>yeast</u> in the crust,
you must take 2 capsules of PROBIOTICS immediately, in
order to prevent any yeast damage to your bowels. Probiotics
will digest and kill the yeast.
If you fail to do that, you may experience pain and bloating.*

Pancakes are Ok, if you eat 2-3, and only with HONEY.

Do not use any syrup, <u>not even Maple syrup</u>, due to the high sugar content (disaccharides), which can damage your bowels.

You can obtain tasty, non pasteurized honey in the health store. A popular brand is: Dutchman`s Gold. 1 Kg is as low as $9.00 plus tax.

GOOD LUCK!

SHEILA BER, 2012.

DISCLAIMER.

Copyright © 2012 Sheila Ber. All rights reserved.

ARTHRITIS HELP and PREVENTION BEST ADVICE.

There are many types of arthritis, ranging from osteoarthritis to rheumatoid arthritis. Osteoarthritis is characterized by the wear and tear of cartilage. Rheumatoid arthritis, on the other hand, is the inflammation of the joints resulting from a viral infection or autoimmune response.

Although the actual cause of arthritis is still not completely known, several potential causes can be due to: injuries, infections, abnormal metabolism, and/or an overactive immune system.

Due to the various causes, treatment programs would therefore focus on the specific causes.

Arthritis common symptoms are: pain, fever, joint stiffness, warmth, redness, and swelling.

Moreover, deformities may result from the limited joint functions. If left untreated, other organs of the body such as the kidneys, heart, and lungs may get affected.

MY BEST ADVICE TO YOU:

The basic causes contributing to Arthritis are as following:

1) High microbial activity that results in inflammation.

Take Probiotics! They have many health benefits, and they help fight and eliminate the microbes, that cause inflammation.

Daily elimination of chemical and microbial toxins! These toxins circulate in your body, impacting your joints negatively, causing inflammation, pain, and swelling. Daily elimination help reduce all these symptoms.

2) Mechanical action of the joints, and cartilage erosion. Cartilage acts as insulation between the bones. Causes vary, and include wear and tear: constant use, overuse or wrong use of the joints, increases the risk of damage to them.

Minimize wearing high heels. Wear comfortable shoes that provide you with an adequate support.
Check also your body balance. Imbalanced body affects the way you walk, and thus affects also the mechanical function of your knees. If you feel that you are lacking balance, see a Chiropractor, or a Physiotherapist. You may need to adjust your back and posture periodically.

*Exercise: Doing daily exercises, within your comfortable limits, with a little challenge or resistance, will help you build endurance, balance, and mobility.

Please see clause #15 (page #49) for further information.

3) Pressure - Exerting pressure from heavy weight, on joints, particularly the knees, can contribute to further damage and erosion of the cartilage, tendons and the bones .Do not carry heavy weights. Handle weight that you feel is light, and that will not exert pressure on your knees.
Your knees carry a large part of your body weight.

If you are overweight, you will benefit greatly from losing weight that feels comfortable to you, and that also will benefit your knees, and other joints.

4) <u>Temperature</u> - Keep your joints warm, especially the knees during cool and cold seasons.

The knees are very sensitive to cold. Cold temperature aggravates and stiffens them, as well as all other joints, resulting in inflammation and pain, particularly if you are already suffering from some degree of Arthritis.
<u>Solution</u>: Wear leg warmers, which can be pulled over your knees, day and night, to ensure that they are kept constantly warm!

*You can obtain Acrylic leg warmers at most Dollarama stores, at a very low price.

Note: Keeping the knees warm, when the temperature of your surrounding is under 15 ∘C, makes a world of a difference, to how your knees feel and act!

5) <u>Moisture</u> - High humidity level in the air, and lower barometric pressure represent unfavourable environment for Arthritic sufferers.

*Take care of your joints, especially the knees, by applying a barrier on the area of the joints.

<u>Solution</u>: A suitable barrier can be any ordinary, healthy cooking oil, such as Grape Seed, Almond, Mustard, or even Canola oil.
Massage daily, any of the above on the joint area, for a few seconds. The oil keeps a layer on the skin, that keeps the moisture out.

Additionally, oils that are rich in Anti-Oxidants, when penetrating the skin, will provide your joints with excellent health benefits, as well as with much needed lubrication.

6) <u>Imbalanced body pH</u>. Your blood and urine pH has to be slightly alkaline, and if it is acidic, it gives rise to higher microbial activity in your body, oxygen deprivation, thus higher inflammation level, that manifests itself in many ways.

Overall body pH has a significant effect on all joints, organs, blood vessels, tissues, hormones, in short, all body systems. Acidic pH is attributed to <u>high</u> consumption of sugars/carbohydrates, proteins, oils and fats, and stress.

<u>To alkalize daily do the following:</u> Take 1/2 tsp Baking Soda (Arm & Hammer) in 1 cup water, with 1 Potassium table 99 mg. You may need to repeat the above 2-3 times a day, so that your body will be slightly alkaline: pH 7.0-7.5.

To test your body pH, you simply test the pH in your urine, as following:
A simple test is done with a Q-Tip (coated with Turmeric, and has light yellow color) and is placed under the stream of urine. If the pH is acidic, it will remain yellow, and if it is alkaline, the color of the Q-Tip will appear in color ranging from orange to red wine.

Orange to red wine, are the colors that you have to obtain. If you see yellow on your Q-tip, immediately, alkalize, by taking your Baking Soda drink, as described above.

**To prepare your Q-Tips for the test, do the following simple steps: In a small container, place several tablespoons of rubbing Ethyl alcohol (S.D.M Pharmacy.). Mix in: 1/2 teaspoon Turmeric powder. Mix well. Immerse 10-20 Q-Tips in the mixture.

Let dry over a piece of paper. Cut them in 1/2, so you can use both ends for more tests. You'll have a month supply to do your daily pH tests.

7) <u>Electrolyte imbalance</u>- If your body electrolyte fluids are not balanced, the electrical conductivity in your joints is not optimal. Thus resulting in less of the following:

blood circulation, oxygen , nutrients and energy.

To balance your electrolytes take daily: Multi-minerals, and also 1 Potassium tablet 99 mg - 1-2x a day.

8) <u>Diet</u> - Diet that consists of excessive sugars, carbohydrates and junk foods that contain also unhealthy oils and fats, that may be harmful and toxic to your joints, and body in general.

Diets high sugars in any form, including carbohydrates (carbs), will feed the anaerobic bacteria and yeast in your body, multiplying them and increasing the microbial level, which will result in inflammation and pain, consequently erosion of joints cartilage, and bones.

Reduce your sugars/carbs intake!

*Note: Honey (monosaccharides) in moderation is good. It breaks down and gets absorbed more rapidly, allowing less time for microbes to feed and multiply.

Honey can be used in coffee, tea, baking, and more. It is kept at room temperature, but has to be handled carefully, by always using clean utensils during usage, to prevent any microbial contamination.

9) <u>Mental state</u> - If you are experiencing stress that is extreme, or if your emotions are fluctuating, out of control. It is individual, and each person extreme varies, according to their coping capabilities.

Find positive ways to deal with it, and do not let it linger, as it is harmful to your health, and your joints will feel it!

Stress converts body pH to acidic as following:

INCREASED STRESS + ACIDIC DIET + TOXINS = INCREASED BODY ACIDITY = LOW ACIDIC pH.

INCREASED ACIDITY = HIGHER MICROBIAL LEVEL.

HIGHER MICROBIAL LEVEL = MORE TOXINS = INCREASED INFLAMMATION AND PAIN!

RELAXATION + SLIGHTLY ALKALINE DIET + TOXIN ELIMINATION = DECREASED BODY ACIDITY = SLIGHTLY ALKALINE pH.

DECREASED ACIDITY = LOWER MICROBIAL LEVEL = BALANCED INTESTINAL FLORA = DECREASED INFLAMMATION AND PAIN! = OPTIMUM HEALTH!

ALKALIZE DAILY!   *See page #41.*

When body pH is very acidic, it impedes normal metabolic activities, resulting in inflammation and pain.

*Body acidity is detected in blood and urine, as well as in saliva.

TO ARREST THE PROGRESSION OF ARTHRITIS IN YOUR JOINTS, take the following daily:

1) GLS-500 - (Glucosamine Sulfate) or GLS-1000, 1 capsule - 2x a day.

You may take GLS with food, if experiencing any discomfort.

*Give it time to have full effect: 3-4 weeks!

2) Boswellia - An anti-inflammatory herb that is very effective. 1 tablet 2x a day.

3) MSM - (Methylsulfonylmethane) 1000 mg. - excellent in reducing pain and inflammation. Take 1 capsule 2x a day. For increased pain and inflammation, you may safely take 1-6 capsules 3x a day, preferably on empty stomach.

4) *Multi-vitamins & minerals.*

5) *B-Complex* - *1 tablet - 1-2x daily, with food, to help with stress.*

6) *Vitamin D3* - *4,000- 6,000 I.U. caplets, 2 times daily, taken with Omega oil/Flax oil for maximum absorption. Vitamin D is an anti-inflammatory steroid.*

It is very beneficial particularly in higher concentration, for keeping inflammation down.

It maintains healthy bones, and balanced Thyroid. Vitamin D3 can be safely taken, up to 10,000 I.U. a day. Improvement in health,
and reduction in inflammation, is noticed immediately.

7) *Beta Carotene* – *10,000 I.U. - 1 caplet 2x a day, with food. When you feel better, gradually reduce to 1 caplet once daily. The vitamin helps to fight inflammation!!!*

Beta Carotene converts to vitamin A, and is stored in the liver.

8) <u>Cod liver oil</u> – *Cod liver oil is highly anti inflammatory, as it high in the following: vitamin A & D, omega 3, EPA and DHA.*

The oil has many health benefits. I cannot emphasize enough, how helpful it is in reducing inflammation and pain in the joints, as well as throughout the body.
Take 2-4 tablespoon liquid oil a day, before or after meals. Cod liver oil also reduces body cholesterol level, helps with clearing inflammation from the lungs, and it alleviates symptoms of depression!

9) *Aspirin - 81 mg <u>coated</u> - even every other day. Take it with food only! It is very effective in reducing inflammation.*

You can verify this by checking your blood ESR (Erythrocyte sedimentation rate) level, when taking a blood test.

10) *Calcium Citrate - This form is more absorbable. Take 1,000 - 1,200 mg a day, along with vitamin C, to aid with absorption, in order to maintain strong bones.*

11) Enzymes *– They promote better metabolism,*
And aid in digestion. Enzyme treatments for curing Arthritis
have by far produced more positive results.

The use of <u>proteolytic enzymes</u> such as Serrapeptase has
shown that these enzymes are capable of dissolving dead or
scar tissues without harming the healthy living tissues.

They are much safer alternative for steroidal and non steroidal
inflammatory drugs such as NSAIDs. They are also considered
<u>a safer option</u> over any exotic treatment.

12) Coenzyme Q10 *– Coenzymes are essential organic*
compounds that attach to enzymes to help them catalyze all
reactions.
Coenzyme Q10 boost the immune system, and helps with the
production of energy.

13) Cherries *– the berries are very helpful in lowering*
inflammation, and they are rich in many vitamins including
vitamin A &C, and also Potassium.

They assist in reducing body acidity. You can have them fresh or in any other form.
Cherry syrup diluted in a 1 glass of water, can be also helpful.

14) Copper bracelet- Copper is believed to have antioxidant properties to prevent free radicals from damaging joints. Copper is gradually absorbed through the skin, relieving pain. You can wear it day and night. It works!

15) Exercise & Yoga - You must exercise daily, 15-20 minutes, to keep your joints, as well as your muscles from getting stiff. If you don't, you will experience poor mobility.

When you mobilize or work your joints and muscles, your body secrets essential biochemical lubricating fluids, gradually helping you to reach optimum mobility.

NOTE: Even if you are experiencing great pain, make your best efforts to exercise. You will only feel better later, as the pain eventually subsides!

Lubricating fluids slowly make it easier to exercise. If you are in extreme pain, you may take Tylenol, 1/2 hour before the workout.

<u>Yoga</u> - Doing yoga even 10-15 minutes a day, lying on your back comfortably, will provide you with many health benefits, physically, mentally, and spiritually.

You can check some of the exercises in the following websites:

<u>http://www.shapefit.com/yoga-exercises-introduction.html</u>

and

<u>http://www.livestrong.com/article/419696-gentle-exercises-when-lying-down/</u>

I hope you find the above information helpful.

SHEILA BER, 2012.

Disclaimer

Copyright © 2012 Sheila Ber. All rights reserved.

COLD - EARLY SIGNS' PREVENTION ADVICE.

Feeling the signs of cold coming on? Arrest it before it gets the best of you. Protect yourself immediately, by simply following my best suggestions as following:

Take for several days until you feel better:

1. Beta carotene - 25,000 I.U. with a tbsp of Flax oil, or with some butter, for better absorption, as it is a fat soluble vitamin. It is also anti inflammatory.

2. Vitamin C - 2,000-4,000 mg. a day. Take 2,000 mg. in AM and the same in PM time.

3. *Cod liver oil* - *2 tablespoon a day. The oil provides you with many health benefits: reducing cholesterol, blood thinning, fortifying the nervous system, reducing inflammation, aiding against depression, enhancing memory, and much more. The oil is very high in vitamin A& D.*

4. *Vitamin B-12* - *Best version that is highly absorbable: METHYLCOBALAMINE) Take 1000-2000 mcg. Daily. It is a must vitamin for strengthening immunity, for increasing energy, for depression, nervous system and much more.*

5. *B-Complex -* *1-2capsules a day, for overall health.*

6. *COLOSTRUM-* *2-3 capsules a day. This is absolutely a must supplement for averting a cold and strengthening your immune system. This product is natural, and is found in the mammary glands. Colostrum contains large numbers of antibodies called "secretory immunoglobulin" (IgA)that help protect the mucous membranes in the throat, lungs, and intestines of the infant.*

When feeling worn down, I recommend to always take Colostrum, the first 3 days of an onset of a cold.

Additionally, take <u>Tylenol</u> 325 mg. 1 tablet, 2x a day, for 1-2 days, as it has arresting effect on colds, due to its anti inflammatory action.

<u>*Alkalize!!!*</u> *– The majority of us have acidic pH, due to an acidic diet, high stress level, biological and chemical toxins and other factors.*

To attain a balanced pH, to just slightly alkaline, we have to alkalize daily. Acidic pH (an imbalance) has many significant negative implications on health. Our immune defence is lowered, and the result is higher microbial level, increased inflammation, causing disease, including the common cold.

<u>*How to alkalize*</u>*: Take ½ tsp Baking Soda (Arm & Hammer brand) in 1 cup water, stir well, and drink along with 1 Potassium tablet 99 mg. Potassium is necessary in order to keep body electrolyte fluids balanced, as well as to maintain normal blood pressure level.*

*Stay away from junk food.

*Reduce sugar intake! (including carbohydrates). *refrain from consuming red meat, as it places a burden
on the immune system, due to longer digestion time.

*Eat fish, or chicken, as these provide more health benefits, and are anti-inflammatory. They help you heal more quickly.

*To rid of phlegm, take Turmeric powder. It will clear your lungs, fairly quickly. Take 1 tbsp in 1 cup boiled water, stir well, cool down, and drink 1/3- 3x a day, until you feel better! Drink it before or after meals. It really works!

*Drink chicken soup, the real one! Commercial packages will not provide you with the same health benefits.

If you don't have chicken soup, eat chicken meat in any form you like, preferably not fried. It can be in a wrap, in a sandwich, or on its own.

*keep your body extremities (head & feet) warm, as they are more sensitive to temperature changes, and can influence your cold symptoms negatively.

I wish you a quick recovery.

SHEILA BER, 2012.

Disclaimer

Copyright © 2012 Sheila Ber. All rights reserved.

SHEILA BER BIOGRAPHY   2012.

Professionally:

I'm a **Microbiological/Chemical Technologist**, currently working as a **Naturopathic consultant**.
I worked in Microbiology and Chemistry, for about 12 years, in the Pharmaceutical, cosmetics, and toiletry industries.

I started out as a microbiological/Chemical Analyst. I Performed: chemical and microbiological analysis of raw materials, finished products, variety of packaging materials and their compatibility with different range of finished products.

Chemical analysis tests were carried out with up to date technologically advanced instruments, such as Spectrophotometers, and other apparatus.
Microbiological tests including incubation of samples, and microscopical studies of a variety of bacteria, yeast, and fungus.

I was also involved in Research & Development, and in formulations of large variety of products.
I've carried out many formulations, and modified some when required.

I've advanced several years later, to a higher position with the title of Quality Control Manager.

My work included:

1) Quality Control of raw materials, finished products, packaging.

2) I was responsible for managing and supporting the laboratory personnel.

3) Additionally, I have carried out inspections on the production floor facilities, the equipment, including ventilation system, and other systems. Monthly reporting on the findings, my recommendations, and implementation of required corrective actions.

4) Communication with Health Canada, particularly to obtain their regulatory approvals for new patents and new products. Providing them with documentation, and MSDS information of the raw material involved, in all the formulations.
I have tremendously enjoyed all the above duties.

It's very technically involved work, very interesting, and challenging.

Personally:

Generally, I'm rather unconventional, though as getting older, I become slightly more conventional. I like things straight, simple, and uncomplicated.
I like helping people. I try to view things, situations, from different perspectives.

I refrain from judging others, but need to know all the facts and reasons for their particular behaviour, thoughts and actions, before forming any opinion.
I take everything with a grain of salt, always stay alert, and cautious.

Life has its highs and lows, but I always try to stay afloat. Trying is the key word!

I often check my expectations, and keep them in perspective.

At the age of 20, I've completed 2 years of service, in the Army, filling the position of Sergeant. It was definitely, a significant lifetime experience for me.

I have two grown up sons. I love them very dearly.
I enjoy being a caring mother, not perfect, and with always
room for improvement.

EDUCATION:
I've graduated with **Honours in Science,** *and with* **Distinction in**
Physics.

Seneca College
Microbiological/Chemical Technology

Technical school
Architecture/Mechanical Drafting

School of Accounting
General Accounting

OCCUPATION:

I'm currently working as a Naturopathic Consultant.

<u>EMPLOYMENT HISTORY:</u>
DRUG TRADING COMPANY - Toronto
Microbiological/Chemical Technologist

FABERGE - Toronto
Quality Control/ Laboratory Manager

REVLON - Toronto
Quality Control/ Laboratory Manager

ACCENTURE Business for Utilities - Toronto
Accounting/Administration

I **Lived in:**

1) Toronto, Canada,
2) Argentina, Buenos Aires.

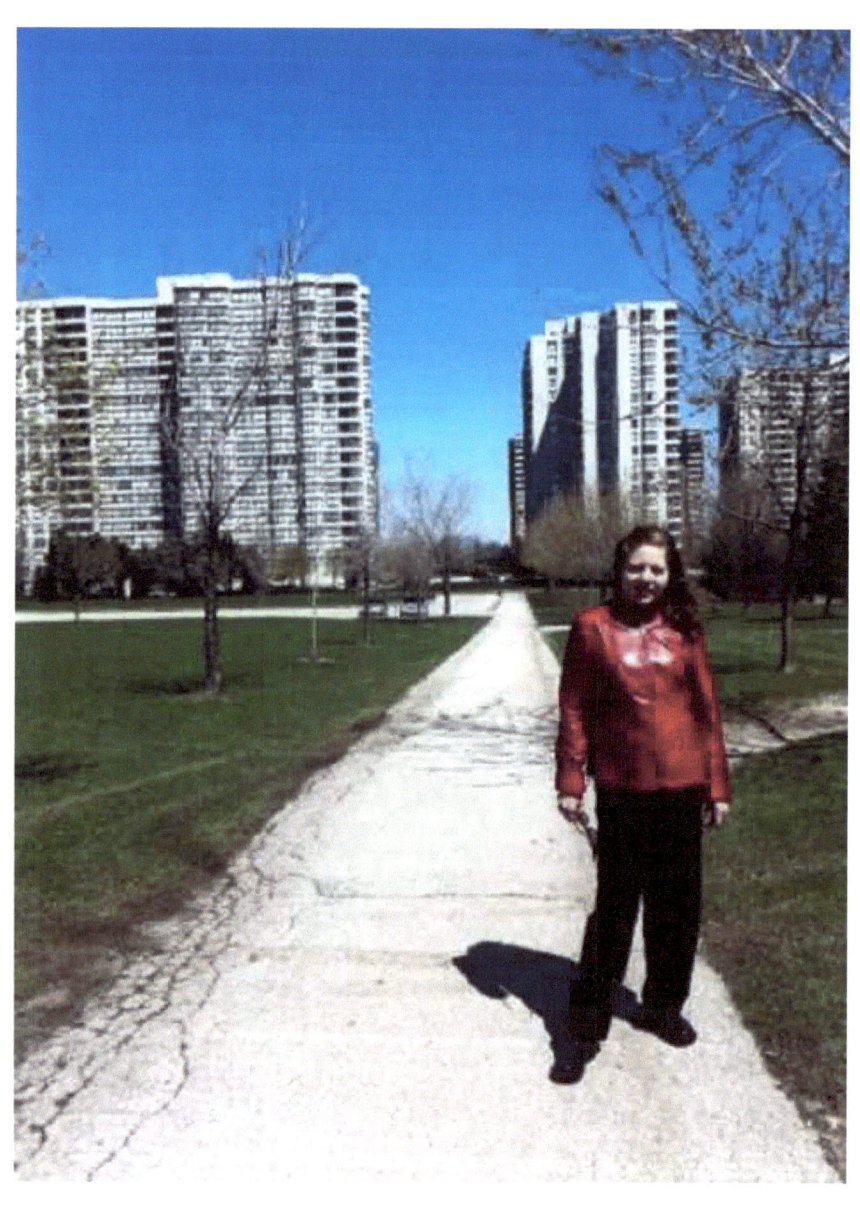

SHEILA BER, 2012.
(SHULLA)

Disclaimer.

Copyright © 2012 Sheila Ber. All rights reserved.

ALKALIZE and SURVIVE!

See "Alkalize & Survive" book by Sheila Ber
at: *www.Amazon.com*
     www.Creatspace.com
     www.Kobobooks.com
     www.Indigo.Chapters.ca

www.ingramcontent.com/pod-product-compliance
Lightning Source LLC
Chambersburg PA
CBHW041505280526
45792CB00004B/1136